I Finally Understand!

I Finally Understand!

✦

A Personal Weight Loss Story

Deb Micinski

iUniverse, Inc.
New York Bloomington Shanghai

I Finally Understand!
A Personal Weight Loss Story

Copyright © 2008 by Deb Micinski

iUniverse books may be ordered through booksellers or by contacting:

iUniverse
1663 Liberty Drive
Bloomington, IN 47403
www.iuniverse.com
1-800-Authors (1-800-288-4677)

Because of the dynamic nature of the Internet, any Web addresses or links contained in this book may have changed since publication and may no longer be valid.

You should not undertake any diet/exercise regimen recommended in this book before consulting your personal physician. Neither the author nor the publisher shall be responsible or liable for any loss or damage allegedly arising as a consequence of your use or application of any information or suggestions contained in this book.

ISBN: 978-0-595-51185-3 (pbk)
ISBN: 978-0-595-61792-0 (ebk)

Printed in the United States of America

This book is dedicated to my family and friends for all their love and support. I love you all!

Contents

Preface

Chances are by reading this book you, like me, have read a number of books, advertisements, magazine articles, etc., on how to lose weight. So I don't want to bore you with a lot of mumbo jumbo you've probably already read before.

My goals for writing this "guide" are simple. I want to provide you with tools and information to help you successfully lose weight and keep it off for the rest of your life! I'll briefly share "my story" and experiences with traditional diets, exercise, etc., but mainly focus on the realistic, common sense approach that finally worked for me as well as the tips, tricks and philosophies I've learned along the way. I'll also discuss the importance of developing a healthy mind and spirit and its vital role in achieving success.

Let me say right up front, I don't claim to have all the answers here. I make no promises nor offer any "money back guarantees". I understand how different we all are, what works for some may not work for others ... but that's precisely why I believe this system works ... it's as individual as you are because *you* make all the choices!

Okay, ready to get started?

Introduction

"How Do You Stay So Skinny?"

"You're probably one of those lucky people with a *"high metabolism"* and never had to worry about your weight, right?"

Boy, if I had a dollar for every time … *well, I think you know where I'm going.*

The truth is I'm not one of those "lucky" people. In fact, over a period of six years I gained over 40 pounds!! Now 40 pounds may not sound like a big deal to someone who is 100+ pounds overweight, but for those of us struggling to lose 20, 30, 40 pounds, etc., it can feel just as challenging, overwhelming and heartbreaking.

While our personal weight loss goals may vary, one goal we all share is learning how to keep the weight off long term. This is where most of us fail, including me until I FINALLY learned how to lose the weight and successfully keep it off *(even after two pregnancies and while going through menopause)* … for over 20 years now!

No, I'm not a doctor, dietician, health care professional, fitness expert or famous talk show host. Nor do I have the luxury of a personal chef or professional fitness trainer "on staff" in my home. I'm your average, 47- year- old middle- class working wife and mother of two teenage children.

I've never written or published anything before, and honestly never even considered the idea until a friend put the idea in my head one day during a conversation about losing weight. I happened to mention how often I have people ask me how I stay thin. My friend somewhat jokingly replied, "Hey, maybe you should write a book!" I chuckled and replied "Yeah, right!" and basically forgot about it.

Several months later I was on my way out of the gym one day when a woman stopped me and asked if she could ask me a few questions. Somewhat puzzled since I didn't know the woman, I curiously agreed.

"I've seen you here before and just wondered if you've ever had a weight problem before? How often do you come to the gym? What do you normally eat? May I ask how old you are?" Our conversation was relatively short, but pleasant, and she seemed genuinely interested in what I had to say.

As I drove home, I thought more about our conversation and how much it reminded me of so many other similar conversations I'd had in the past ... and then I remembered what my friend said several months earlier about writing a book.

A BIG smile slowly crossed my face.

Wow! Just the mere thought of doing something like that ... I mean ... ME write a book!?! Ha, that's crazy!

Well, time passed, but for some reason this crazy idea of writing a book never seemed to. It's sort of hard to explain, but *"situations"* seemed to keep popping up in my daily life "reminding" me in some strange way that I needed to write this book ... *"signs"* perhaps!? Who knows? But, I do know I contemplated the idea for well over a year until finally deciding one day to just do it!

So, three years later, here we are.

You may be asking, "Three years?! This is a short book, what took me so long?" Well, in addition to being an inexperienced writer, finding time to work on it was a real challenge sometimes with work, family and household responsibilities.

Through it all though I have to say I've been most impressed *(and surprised)* by my persistence to stick with it until it was finished. I mean, I could have quit any-time. I always had a good excuse. Plus, I never told anyone I was writing it so no one was holding me accountable. But for some inexplicable reason, I felt it was "important" in some way that I finish it.

So, here it is, FINALLY, from me to you.

1

My Short Story

Now my story may be a little different from others you may have read. I was not a fat kid. I never weighed 200+ pounds. I never suffered from anorexia or bulimia. My battle with weight didn't actually begin until I was about 20 years old and started dieting to lose ten pounds.

I was a very active teenager and participated in a variety of sports including gymnastics, softball, volleyball and bowling. At 5 foot 4 1/2 inches tall and 105 pounds, I ate whatever I wanted and never gained a pound. Obviously, no weight problem here, right? Well, there wasn't until after I graduated from high school and began working full time as a clerical assistant. My lifestyle changed significantly. I now sat behind a desk all day, stopped participating in physical sports *(except bowling)*, but continued to eat as I always had.

Within a few months I began to notice a lot of my clothes were fitting rather tight … some didn't fit at all! I suspected I'd gained some weight, but honestly didn't think too much about it until I had to make a routine visit to the doctor's office. I stepped on the scale to be weighed and to my surprise or better yet, SHOCK, my suspicions were confirmed. Yes, I had indeed gained weight. Twelve pounds to be exact! I was stunned! Twelve pounds! How did this happen?!

Well, there was no doubt in my mind what I had to do … I had to lose it! The question was, how? Suddenly trapped in unfamiliar territory, I didn't know the first thing about losing weight.

I had to get educated … FAST!

Now, okay I know what you're thinking. Sure, I gained twelve pounds but I still only weighed 117 pounds, right? So, what's the big deal? Okay, well keep in mind I was 20 years old and … I GAINED TWELVE POUNDS! To a typical young female this was a HUGE deal! In fact, it turned out to be a critical turning point in my life.

Almost overnight, I was drawn to anything and everything that had to do with losing weight. The latest "fad diets", popular diet books, magazine ads, television ads, etc., etc. I'm sure you know the ones I'm talking about … big, bold headlines that read, **"Drop 20 Pounds in Two Weeks"**, **"Watch Fat Melt Away Overnight With This New Miracle Pill"**, **"Lose 50 Pounds and Still Eat Anything You Want"**, etc. There's an endless array of products, pills and diet plans out there that claim they'll "help" you lose weight, and whether we like to admit it or not, when you're eager to lose weight, ads like this do get our attention.

With consumer demand today for products and services that offer quick satisfaction/gratification, we can't help but be seduced by ads using terms like "rapid", "overnight", "miracle", etc., especially when they're combined with "easy", "effortless", etc.

Like it or not, most of us are easy prey. Especially when you're inexperienced like I was, or have reached the point of desperation. You may begin reading the ad skeptical, but as you continue reading all the success stories, promises and guarantees of quick, huge weight loss, you can't help but think how great it would be if it worked that way for you and you could lose 10, 20, 30 pounds or more. Just think how great you'd look for the holidays, the family wedding, your high school reunion, or that tropical vacation you're planning!

Now they've got you!

Let's be honest, most of us will purchase just about anything if it offers us an *opportunity* to lose weight … regardless of whether we truly believe it will work or not.

For example:

ATTENTION … ATTENTION … Newly discovered fat burning pill allows you to eat anything you want and lose 25 pounds in just two short weeks!!

Wow! Lose 25 pounds in just two weeks! Sounds great doesn't it? But given what you may already know about losing weight, do you honestly believe this will *realistically* work?

If we logically think about it, the answer would be "No", right? But losing weight for most of us is a very emotional issue, so decisions and/or choices we make are more likely based on our emotional state at the time ... it doesn't really matter if they make logical sense or not.

When we feel desperate and *desire* to believe, we can convince ourselves of almost anything, can't we? What if this is the "ONE" ... the one that will finally work for me? What if it really does work the way they say it does and I could lose 25, 30 or even 50 pounds by the time I _____. *I'm sure you can fill in the blank.* Do I risk passing up this *opportunity*?

But what if it doesn't work?

Hey, even if it doesn't work, I'm not really out much. I mean, isn't $39.95 a small price to pay for the chance to be 25 pounds thinner in just two weeks? Excited by the possibility, you reach for the phone, dial the 800 number and place your order.

Okay, so now what? What do you do in the meantime while you're waiting to receive your "miracle in the mail"?

Well ... S P L U R G E, of course! Silly!

Hey, come on! If you're like me, you've just opened the door to a *guilt-free* opportunity to eat all the stuff you wouldn't normally eat. So, why not indulge and eat that hot fudge sundae, bacon cheeseburger, french fries and slice of cheesecake. After all, according to the ad, you'll quickly lose anything you gain in the interim anyway once you start their program, right?

Sound familiar?

Chances are the only thing you'll actually lose is your $39.95 *(plus shipping)*! Obviously, I'm speaking from personal experience here, but I'm sure I'm not alone.

So, I guess the question is why do we do this? Why do we continue to spend our hard earned dollars on products like these when we've had no real success with them in the past?

Sure, we want to lose weight, but is that always the only reason?

Maybe you never really thought about this … I know I didn't. At the time, I was completely convinced my motive was purely to lose weight. Boom! No question! But when I look back now, I honestly think there were times when I just became so tired of constantly having the burden of losing weight on my mind, I embraced any opportunity to free myself from it for a while. Purchasing these products provided me the *excuse* I felt I needed to temporarily shift the responsibility/burden on to someone/something else so I could take a break!

Did you ever purchase a weight loss book (or other) only to let it sit on a shelf for days or weeks because you can't seem to "find the time" (or procrastinate for other reasons) to read it? During this time of procrastination, do you feel less guilty about indulging? What was the motivating factor at the time for purchasing the book? To make you feel better in some way … band-aid feelings of guilt, obligation or responsibility? Why can't you seem to find time to read it? Is it possible once you've read it you'll feel obligated to take action and you're enjoying this period of freedom and guilt free indulgence?

Believe me … I *desperately* wanted to lose weight. I just couldn't stick to any of the diet plans I tried long term. I'd always end up quitting and repeat the same cycle over and over again … diet, lose weight, quit, binge, gain weight, feel bad/guilty, start another diet, lose weight, quit, binge, gain, guilty, diet, lose, quit, binge, gain, etc., etc. Aaahhh! It's shear madness when you stop and think about it, isn't it?

Eventually, I learned that each time I "handed over" the responsibility/control for losing weight to someone/something else I just set myself up to fail again. Why? Because I wasn't truly taking personal responsibility! I was passing the buck! I had to stop this cycle of behavior and dependency on the other guy's easy, quick fix solutions to lose weight and make a commitment once and for all to use realistic, healthy methods to lose weight. There were no shortcuts!!

Sure, this all makes sense to me now, but I'm hard headed (*I know my family finds that hard to believe*) and I have to learn EVERYTHING the hard way. Finding the right way to lose weight was no exception. In the next chapter, I discuss some of the dieting craziness I went through over the years until I finally understood this.

So, let the madness begin …

2

Losing it! (Literally)

As mentioned earlier, in an effort to lose the twelve pounds I gained, I, like most people decided I had to go on a diet. My first diet of choice was a popular "fad diet" at that time, the infamous Grapefruit Diet. I can't say I really remember too much about it, other than eating a lot of grapefruit! Well, it didn't take long before I had my fill of grapefruit and canker sores, and quit that diet!

Not to be deterred, I tried another one … then another … and another. With each fad diet I tried, I'd lose some weight initially, but could never stay on one long enough to lose all the weight. Worse yet, each time I went off a diet, I'd eat everything in sight for days. Consequently, I regained any weight I struggled so hard to lose and many times even gain a few more pounds!

As twisted as it sounds, I felt allowing myself the freedom to eat anything I wanted after I quit a diet was sort of my "reward" for having deprived my self so long from the foods I loved.

Once I realized the fad diets weren't going to be the answer, I began searching for other options. I tried calorie counting … you know the 1,200–1,500 calorie a day thing. Again, it initially worked, but the weight loss was too slow. Impatient and wanting faster results, I lowered my calorie intake to just 500 calories a day. Well, it didn't take long before I quit that diet too … due to starvation!!

Over a period of about two years, I was on and off a number of different diets. What did I gain? Well, fifteen more pounds to be exact! Now instead of just twelve pounds to lose, I had 27!

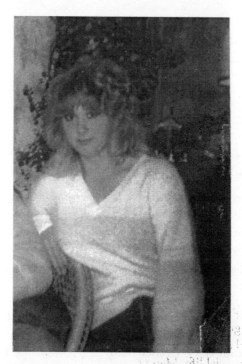

This is a picture of me taken Thanksgiving, 1982. I was 22 years old and weighed 132 pounds. Don't you love the hair?!

Convinced I just hadn't found the right "fix" yet my search continued for the latest, greatest, new fangled "scientific breakthrough" product or diet that was finally going to be the answer to my prayers.

As we all know, products like this aren't hard to find. Just pick up any magazine, turn on television or do a search for diets, weight loss, etc., on the Internet and you'll be inundated with choices. Just for kicks, the next time you see a weight loss ad on television, challenge yourself to find the small printed statement, "Results Not Typical" (*it generally shows up at some point in most ads*).

My question is, "If the advertised weight loss is not 'typical' then how much is typical?" Isn't that what we really want to know? Hey, I don't care about the "rare" or "unusual" cases ... I want to know what the average person can lose!

The other thing I always found interesting with most weight loss products I purchased was the "recommended diet" to use in conjunction with their product.

So wait a minute ... if I do lose weight is it because of their product or the recommended diet? Hmmm!

Okay ... I digress! Let's move on ...

Since none of the weight loss products I purchased had worked for me, I decided it was time to try a more "common sense" approach. So, I bought one of those popular diet plan books written by a doctor ... you know the ones I'm talking about. Boy was it thick! (*My goal was to start losing weight today, not months from now*). After a few days of reading stuff I already knew (*and a lot of scientific mumbo jumbo I didn't really understand or care about*), I skipped through it until I found the chapter that discussed the actual diet plan. I reviewed the sample menus and recipes, made my grocery list and off to the store I went.

I also joined a local fitness center and started exercising regularly.

I was doing great! I diligently followed the plan and exercised regularly for about three weeks and *Voila!* I lost ten pounds. I was thrilled! However, the downside was I was quickly growing tired of the restricted food choices I had and worse yet, feeling like a social outcast with my friends! Like most single people in their 20's, I had a very active social life. Many times that included eating out and sometimes late at night, which of course is a "no-no" on just about any diet. So, I'd occasionally cheat. After all, if a guy asked me out to dinner, I wasn't about to tell him I was on a diet! Come on ... I might as well wave a big red flag asking, "Hey buddy, did you get a look at the size of my butt?"

Needless to say, it didn't take long before my *occasional* cheating became *frequent* cheating. Eventually I reverted right back to my old eating habits again and quickly regained the weight I'd lost and ... even more in the months and years that followed.

Jumping ahead to age 24, I now weighed 142 pounds!

Quite frankly, I was completely lost! The whole situation felt totally out of my control and I didn't know how to get a handle on it.

Defeated and incapable of losing weight on my own, I decided to turn to the *experts* for help and called a local weight loss center.

On the day of my appointment, I was to meet with one of their representatives in a conference room. As I walked in, the representative looked up, gave me the "once over" and said in a somewhat sarcastic tone, "What are YOU doing here?" *(The implication was she didn't think I was FAT enough to be there).*

Now, you would think that should have made me feel kind of good, right? WRONG! It honestly made me feel as though I would not be taken seriously... and believe me, I was very serious!

Despite the representative's attitude, I did join.

The center recommended members purchase their products and weekly supply of diet aids, e.g., protein powders, etc., in addition to certain grocery store items *(altogether I think it cost me about $50 a week)*. I followed their weight loss program for about six weeks and lost about fifteen pounds. Great! Right?

Well, it was. But once again, it was a challenge to stick to with my social life. On top of that, it was expensive! With my small salary, it didn't take long before I just couldn't afford to stay on the program any longer and had to quit. As always, slowly but surely, I regained all the weight I'd lost.

While we've discussed some of the diets I've tried, below are some other ways I tried to lose weight over the years.

Exercise: Yes, but early on it was only when I was also dieting. Even then it was inconsistent. I'd go weeks or months without exercising at all then have periods when I'd exercise everyday ... sometimes with such intensity it was as though I was trying to lose all the weight in a single workout! Working out like this just left me in pain and hating it!

Diet drinks/shakes: I'm sure you know what I'm talking about here. Sorry, but I don't consider *drinking* anything a meal! First of all, there's no chewing and chewing to me equates eating! Never mind the fact, I was always hungry again an hour or two later.

Diet Pills: Yes, I tried these. I took them as recommended and they did curb my appetite, but boy was I nasty! I believe they've improved these over the years, but the diet pills of yester-year just left me feeling shaky and irritable. I had to stop taking these regularly or I think my family would have kicked me out of the house!

Fasting: Do I even need to explain why this didn't work?

As you can see, I've tried a number of ways to lose weight over the years, but none of them were successful long term. Consequently, my weight was up and down like a yoyo. By the time I was 26 years old, I weighed 148 lbs. Now, depending on your situation, 148 pounds may be good thing. But understand my situation ... I GAINED OVER 40 POUNDS! I'm sure you can understand why I would be be upset about that!

But honestly, I was beyond just being upset; I was devastated! I remember thinking if I only had some *willpower* I would have lost this weight by now.

What was wrong with me?!

To make matters worse, I'd also been "binge" eating *(I think we are all familiar with this term)*. This alone significantly contributed to my weight gain. On the way home after a late night out with friends, I'd stop at a fast food restaurant *(sometimes two in a night),* order a bunch of junk food, wolf it down and then go home to bed.

Occasionally, I even resorted to taking laxatives as a desperate attempt to rid my body of all the food I ate. It was crazy!

Looking back now, I believe I was at my lowest point during this time. I can remember times of shoveling food in my mouth and crying at the same time. I knew I was hurting myself, but in some twisted way believed I deserved this "punishment". I now understand just how emotionally and physically self-destructive this behavior is.

Alone, angry and depressed, I remember how envious I was of pretty, thin women. In my mind, they had life made. They could have anything they wanted, and didn't even realize it. When I looked in the mirror, I felt nothing but disgust and worthlessness. I HATED my body! I also hated doing anything that brought attention to my weight. Shopping for clothes was especially tough.

Don't misunderstand, I loved all the cute, trendy clothes I saw the skinny girls wear and when I found them in my size I'd get very excited to try them on. Unfortunately, once I had them on, any excitement usually turned to disappointment because they never looked as good on my body.

Consequently, I usually left the store with nothing but deepened feelings of inadequacy and self-hatred.

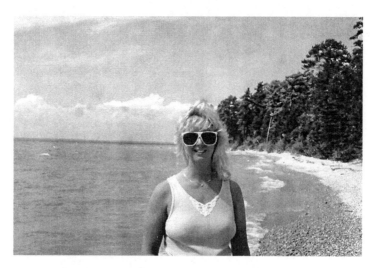

This picture was taken in June, 1987 at Mackinaw Island. I was 26 years old and weighed 148 pounds. Yeah, I know the glasses are hideous aren't they? But it was the 80's and believe it or not these were in style!

3

The lights are on ...
and someone is FINALLY home!

In 1987, I began dating a guy I'd casually known since I was sixteen years old. I'd dated a few other guys (some good, some bad) but he was different. We really felt "connected" right from the start. I loved spending time with him. I was happy and for the first time in years, I didn't feel consumed with issues/anxiety about my weight. I guess I was so preoccupied with actually *living* and *loving* life for a change, I didn't even realize I'd stopped binge eating until weeks later. The funny thing was this renewed *"zest for life"* had nothing to do with my weight ... because my weight hadn't changed.

Several months later, however, I was pleasantly surprised to discover I had lost weight. I think it was only about five or six pounds, but the point was ... I had not been trying to lose weight!

That's when the "lights" finally came on!

Why was I able to lose weight now without even trying? Priding myself on self-discipline, I felt I should have been able to get this weight thing under control a long time ago. So, what's different now? What was I doing wrong before? Curious, I had to dig deeper to find some answers.

I began reviewing the past events of my life, making comparisons of my life then versus today. Surprisingly, it didn't take too long to discover what the real source of the problem was. It was the way I FELT (*emotionally/spiritually*) about myself and my life then. I suddenly realized just how truly unhappy and discontent I was at different times back then. The truth is my *spirit* was broken. The question was, Why? I've always been blessed with a wonderful, supportive family and fantastic friends, so what caused me to feel this way and why wasn't I able to get control of it and "fix it"?!

Well, I gave this a lot of thought and I came to the conclusion, I thought I was trying to fix it … each and every time I started a new diet!

You see, I was so convinced my weight was the sole reason for my unhappiness, I virtually ignored other issues going on in my life and the effect they were having on me.

I honestly believed if I could just lose weight, it would fix everything. I'd have everything I wanted and finally feel free to be happy. Since I repeatedly failed to do that, I didn't feel *worthy* of happiness because I hadn't *earned* that right yet.

Sound familiar?

While there were other contributing factors, *(which I'll get into later)*, the constant failure to lose weight perpetuated a very poor self-image and lack of self-respect. The lack of self-respect triggered the binge eating. The binge eating caused me to gain even more weight. Gaining more weight deepened my feelings of worthlessness and depression.

What a self-destructive cycle! Needless to say, I was an emotional mess!

Time for a fresh start!

As mentioned earlier, after dating ten months or so, I felt happier and better about myself than I had in years. I decided to go back to the gym and start working out again. This time, however, my goals were going to be different. This time it was part of my goal to create a new healthy *lifestyle.*

I vowed to never go on another restrictive diet again! I was going to respect my body and make a commitment to eat healthy and treat my body well from now on. I was also going to take steps to strengthen my mental/spiritual health as well.

Less than 5 months later, I *painlessly* dropped 35 pounds and weighed 113 pounds.

Did I stop eating all the foods I like? No, of course not, I had the "bad stuff" now and then, but focused on eating well most of the time. I also learned some important tricks along the way to help me stay on track that I'll share with you later.

I think you would agree, what we choose to eat is more often out of habit than anything else. So, I knew I had to change my eating habits. But I also knew it couldn't be an "all or nothing" approach because that never worked for me in the past. I had to come up with a plan that was not only realistic but flexible enough to fit my lifestyle.

So, after some analysis, here's what I decided to do:

Since my normal work week was fairly routine compared to my weekends, I focused on eating healthy, watched portion sizes and exercised regularly (3–4 times) during the week. On the weekends, however, I was *allowed* to eat a few "extras" as well as choose whether or not to exercise. Now understand, that doesn't mean I went crazy on the weekends, lying around eating nothing but junk food, etc. It means if I did go out with friends, it was okay to have a couple slices of pizza or an ice cream cone, etc., as long as I stayed in control (*realistic portion sizes)* and continued to eat healthy otherwise.

But come Monday, I MUST return to eating healthy again and exercising regularly. (*Obviously, if you stick to eating healthy and exercising on the weekends too that's even better and a great goal to strive for).*

Wow! This worked! Simply allowing myself the choice/option to have what I wanted occasionally on the weekends made such a difference. It fit into my social life, I didn't feel guilty or deprived and best of all … I was losing weight!

Now I'd be lying if I said I never lost it occasionally and grabbed the chocolate chip cookies, peanut butter, chocolate cake, etc., etc., … old habits are hard to break you know! But honestly, as time went on those weak moments became less and less. When I did have a weak moment, it was generally because it was "that time of the month" or my routine was messed up for some reason.

Eventually it just became a habit to pick the good stuff over the bad. Believe it or not, I even reached the point where sometimes just the thought of how bad something was for me was enough reason to turn it down and choose something healthier. Yes … REALLY!

My self-esteem soared. Not only did I feel great, I was in control.

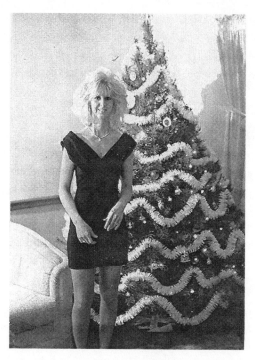

This picture was taken at Christmas, 1988 (about a year and a half after the Mackinaw picture was taken). I was 28 years old and weighed about 112 pounds.

"NOTHING TASTES AS GOOD AS BEING THIN FEELS"

4

Come on … Think Positive!

I believe it is extremely important to recognize how our subconscious thoughts, feelings and attitude can affect *(positively or negatively)* our spirit/self-image and overall life experience. *In my opinion, successfully losing weight depends as much on having a healthy mind/spirit as it does on having a healthy diet/lifestyle.*

I would guess many of us are guilty of focusing more attention on the things we do wrong or haven't accomplished yet than on the things we do right and have accomplished so far in our lives. In our constant drive to succeed, we generally don't take time to fully acknowledge and/or appreciate the goals we've accomplished along the way. However, the opposite tends to be true if we should fail to meet a goal. We can mentally beat ourselves up for days, weeks, months or even years … in some cases, never forgiving ourselves for certain failures.

Unfortunately, we truly can be our own worst enemy sometimes.

The fact is, whether it's in your control or not, sometimes we will succeed and other times we will fail. But it's important to recognize how you're *reacting* to these times of perceived failures. Without a somewhat positive, forgiving attitude, you could be putting yourself on the road to low self-esteem and a poor self-image.

Now, I consider myself to be a positive, upbeat person, who doesn't give up easily *(just ask my husband)*. So I hate to use words like failed, failure, etc., but like most people, I've had my share of perceived failures in life. Belief in the notion "failure is not an option", I was mentally tough on myself when I didn't meet a goal, e.g., losing weight. But when I finally woke up and realized reacting this way wasn't accomplishing anything except destroying my self-esteem, I knew I had to make some important changes.

It took time, practice and discipline, but eventually I learned to focus more on what I gained/learned from each effort or experience rather than on whether I succeeded or failed. Once I started doing this, I quickly discovered I usually learned more during those times of perceived failures than I did when I succeeded anyway. So, I decided I couldn't really consider them failures if I actually learned something, right? With failure comes knowledge?! (*I think someone actually said this, didn't they?*) Equally important, I learned to be *grateful* for each experience in my life.

To put it simply ... you can *choose* to focus on the negative aspects of a situation or you can choose to focus on the positive ones! It's really just that simple and it's in your control!

Let me give you an example. Let's assume for a moment you went on yet another diet/weight loss program and quit before you lost all the weight you wanted (*probably the reason you're reading my book*). Okay, so how do you *choose* to react to this perceived failure? Do you kick yourself while you're down ..."I failed again! I'm such a loser!" ... and inhale a gallon of ice cream?

Or do you choose to look at what you learned/gained from the experience?

Maybe you discovered a great new recipe or a new fruit/vegetable you liked but would have otherwise never tried. Maybe you took an aerobics class and actually enjoyed it! Maybe you met some new people at the gym and expanded your social circle.

Maybe ... the only thing you learned was that you'll never go on that type of diet again! Ha! Now, I may joke, but my point is, even though you may have "failed" to stay on the diet and lose the weight you wanted, you probably still learned something from the effort/experience.

Sure you're disappointed you didn't lose the weight you intended, but why waste time beating yourself up over it? Seriously! What do you gain by doing that? If the truth be told, the diet was probably too restrictive and/or unrealistic anyway and doesn't work for the majority of people who go on it. So, chalk it up to a learning experience, use the knowledge you gained to make better choices and decisions in the future and move on. By looking at the glass "half-full" instead of "half-empty", you'll maintain a positive outlook, gain greater self-confidence and remain mentally strong to take on future challenges.

Okay, here's a slightly different example ...

How do people react when you've told them you're on a diet? Do they congratulate you? Probably not! The truth is they probably feel sorry for you. Why? Because we all know what it means to be on a typical diet ... food restrictions, deprivation and social limitations ... all negative, right?

But how do you think people would react if you told them you were working out and eating healthy? Odds are you'd receive a more favorable *(positive)* reaction. Why? Because we all know working out and eating healthy are key to achieving good health *(positive)*. But more importantly, wouldn't you feel better using this approach instead of forcing yourself to adhere to some restrictive diet?

Obviously, losing weight in itself is generally considered to be a positive thing, but what do you think your chances of success are if you're using a method you truly feel negative about?

Personal experience tells me not too good.

Hopefully, you understand the point I'm trying to make here as I don't want to bore you by belaboring this issue. Let me just sum it up by saying, strive to replace negative thoughts, attitude and behavior with positive ones everyday and you'll be happier and overall more successful in life because of it. Trust me!

Here are a few suggestions to help you get started on a positive track:

- If you're still beating yourself up over some past situation(s), STOP IT! Let it go! Forgive yourself now and recognize what you've learned from it and move on! We are human and we've all done things we may not be too proud of in our lives. It's time to put the stake in the sand, and say ENOUGH! It's time to move on!

- Give yourself permission to be happy right now ... TODAY! Go outside and tell the world ... "I deserve to be happy and I'm choosing to live a happier, healthier life from this day forward!" You owe it to yourself!

- Stop hiding! For those of you doing this, you know exactly what I'm talking about here. Free yourself from self-imposed restrictions! Get out there! Get involved! Let yourself go to be free and start living and enjoying life. Life is meant to be abundant! Start experiencing it!

- Find ways to reduce/eliminate negative thoughts, attitude and behavior in your life. Someone told me once to place a rubber band on my wrist and snap it when I was thinking or acting negative or self-defeating. But if you prefer a less *painful* method, try replacing negative thoughts with thoughts that bring a smile to your face.

Start and continue to make choices in life that are good for <u>YOU</u>!

- Surround yourself with positive, upbeat, supportive people that make you feel good about life. Wean yourself away from negative people as soon as possible, or at the very least, severely limit your time with them.

- Find ways to spend more time doing the things you enjoy … things that make you feel good.

- Challenge yourself to explore new things. Take a class at your local college and/or take up a new hobby you've been interested in but never took the time to pursue.

- Plan little outings, trips or events often so you have something fun and positive to look forward to regularly.

- Finally, be grateful! Take time everyday to acknowledge and appreciate the positive things in your life.

You know, "Take time to smell the roses!"

LIKE SUCCESS, FAILURE IS MANY THINGS TO MANY PEOPLE. WITH POSITIVE MENTAL ATTITUDE, FAILURE IS A LEARNING EXPERIENCE, A RUNG ON THE LADDER, A PLATEAU AT WHICH TO GET YOUR THOUGHTS IN ORDER AND PREPARE TO TRY AGAIN.
—*W. Clement Stone*

5

Spirit

I'm sure we've all heard the saying, "You have to fix what's happening on the *inside* before you can fix what's happening on the *outside.*" Well, from personal experience I found this to be absolutely true. It's really common sense though isn't it? Successfully losing weight *(or anything really)* has to be harder if you're already mentally and/or emotionally stressed out due to other underlying issues in your life.

Unfortunately, some people go years *(even a lifetime)* without ever realizing or addressing the true source(s) of their unhappiness. Preoccupied by issues on the *surface* i.e., their weight, physical appearance, etc., they never look any deeper. Left unaddressed, those underlying problems could be the reason they can't find happiness, lose weight or achieve success in other areas of their life.

Without getting too philosophical, I don't believe, as a society, we're taught to focus enough attention on our inner *(emotional)* feelings or spirit. Conversely, we are taught to focus a great deal of attention to our external *(physical)* appearance. To some degree, I guess it's understandable considering we are literally faced with it everyday.

Each day as we prepare to go out in the world, we look in the mirror and we're confronted once again with the things we dislike about our appearance ... my thighs are too fat, my butt is too big, my nose is crooked, etc., etc. Let's face it, *(no pun intended)* we all understand the way we look can affect how we are treated in the world and how we are judged by our peers. So, it's no surprise why we are more consumed with issues of how we *look* as opposed to how we *feel.*

I was so preoccupied with my appearance *(my weight)*, I overlooked what was really causing me to feel depressed and unhappy. It took being in a good relationship to wake up and realize my weight was not the sole reason for my unhappiness *(because remember I was still overweight)*, I was *spiritually* unhappy with myself and my life! Consequently, I wasn't mentally and/or emotionally strong enough to handle the added stress and challenge of successfully losing weight … it actually just made matters worse.

The reality is, most of us are so busy just trying to keep up with our daily responsibilities of kids, school, work, family, friends, etc., etc., we ignore or don't feel we have time to focus on our emotional needs or spiritual health. Other times, it may just be we don't want to confront those issues that make us feel bad. They may be too painful or difficult to deal with so we continue to push those feelings down.

Unfortunately, as you may know, constantly ignoring and pushing the negative feelings down won't make them go away. Many times, you just end up with *displaced* anger and/or depression. The reality is we all end up dealing with those buried feelings at some point in our lives anyway, whether it's mentally, emotionally or physically through health problems. Many times we never make the connection that the problems we're dealing with today may be a direct result of those unresolved problems of our past … or even present.

Sure, as I look back now, it's easy to see the chain of events that lead to my unhappiness and depression. I just didn't "see" it at the time.

In short, I was attending college full-time and working part-time. I was financially broke and physically exhausted most of the time trying to keep up with school, work and my social life. My relationship ended with my boyfriend of over four years after he confessed he'd become romantically involved with a female co-worker. A married friend, unhappy in his marriage, expressed a romantic interest in me that soon became an obsessive, stalking situation. My car was vandalized four times. My younger sister and brother were both planning their weddings, whereas my life consisted of partying, bar hopping, and bad dates.

Sure, there were other contributing factors, but I don't think it's necessary to go into everything in my past for you to understand the point I'm trying to make. In short, I blamed my weight for all the unhappiness I felt in my life and virtually ignored the effect these other issues were having on me.

These *"other issues"* are what I believe triggered the binge eating. I was looking for something (food) to fill the emotional emptiness I felt.

I know … I know … I hate even saying this because it sounds so cliché. But, honestly for me, even though the bar life had been a lot of fun in my past, as I grew older it only left me feeling emotionally empty and alone.

This is why I recommend you take an honest, hard look at what's going on in your life and address any issues that could be creating stress and/or depression before you make any other attempts to lose weight. If you don't, you could just be setting yourself up for disappointment.

Do you feel in control of your life or do you allow other people or life's issues to control it?

While we should all feel in the "driver's seat" when it comes to making decisions and choices in our lives, this just isn't the case for some people. They become so weighed down by negative issues in their lives, they just don't have the strength or "know how" to pull themselves out of it to gain control again. If you're one of these people, you probably already know allowing this to go on too long can have a huge negative impact on your life, spirit and self-image.

So, if you don't feel in control the way you want to be, start taking steps to get there! As a suggestion you could start by making a list of significant issues in your life right now. (*I find this exercise helpful to bring awareness and perspective to the forefront*). On a sheet of paper, make two columns. In the first column, list the positive things in your life. Things that make you feel good, i.e., people close to you, things you've accomplished and acquired in life that you're proud of, things you enjoy doing, interests, hobbies, etc.

In the second column, list the negatives. Things that make you feel angry, sad, depressed and/or embarrassed, i.e., people, relationships, finances, job, other circumstances, etc.

When you're done, review the positive items first. Take time to really think about each one. Recognize and appreciate the way they make you feel.

Next review the negative column. For each item listed, ask yourself why it makes you feel sad, out of control, and/or embarrassed, etc. Is there something you could or should do to change that situation and/or help improve it? If so, write it down next to that item. While there may be some things you feel are out of your control right now, there may be others you can start doing something about.

(Many times we already know what changes are necessary to correct a bad situation, it's taking action to make those changes that's the hardest).

Keep this list and review/update it daily/weekly. Use it as your "self-help guide" to stay focused on making positive changes as well as a reminder of the wonderful things you already have going on in your life. As changes and improvements are made, goals are achieved, negative items eliminated, etc., update your list. By maintaining focus on the positive things in life, and continuing to take steps to rid yourself of the negatives, it will help you begin to take control of your life again. You'll feel empowered!

Okay, what if this all just sounds good, but everything in your life just seems too overwhelming to deal with?

Well, maybe you should consider some sort of counseling. Now, wait! Let me explain! I know counseling seems to be everyone's "token" advice to someone trying to cope with a difficult time in their life. But please don't dismiss the idea without at least some consideration, especially if you've never tried it. Many times people discover speaking with a professional counselor *(stranger)* is surprisingly easier than anticipated. You also have the assurance of knowing what you discuss is confidential. So, you don't have to worry about family and/or friends finding something out you don't want them to. Also, keep in mind a professional counselor has probably already helped others in the same and/or similar situation you're in, so you should never feel judged or embarrassed.

Whether you seek help/guidance from a professional counselor, doctor, spiritual counselor/leader, friend, etc., doesn't matter. What does matter is taking ACTION! Find a way to release the negative feelings you may be holding on to that are preventing you from living the life of happiness you deserve.

It will take some time and effort … but you WILL get through whatever the issues are as long as you stay committed.

On a personal note: It truly upsets me to watch people live their lives depressed and unhappy simply because they believe only "weak" people resort to counseling, etc. Personally, I see it as the opposite. I believe it takes great strength and character to take responsibility for your actions and attitude and do whatever is necessary to improve your life and the lives of those around you. In my opinion, the weak ones are those who sit back, do nothing and continue to make life miserable for themselves and everyone around them.

The fact is, we all have and/or will be faced with difficult times in our lives, but we have a choice deciding how we'll get through them.

When faced with the challenge of crossing a violent river, do you risk drowning by wading through the rough, choppy water or use the bridge nearby to help you reach the other side safely and easily?

Again, please, please don't be afraid or embarrassed to seek help/guidance if you need it … it's the responsible thing to do and you owe it to yourself and those around you.

YOUR THOUGHTS AND FEELINGS CREATE YOUR LIFE!

6

The Dreaded "E" Word

Come on now … you knew it was coming!

I feel so strongly about this subject I had to devote a separate chapter to it. So, please don't skip it! It's really important to read if you're truly serious about losing weight.

Now, I know some people hate to keep hearing about the "E" word—Exercise. But I honestly don't know how anyone can successfully lose weight and keep it off long term without incorporating some kind of regular exercise in their life. Now, that doesn't mean you have to become a fitness fanatic! However, I do firmly believe we all need to include regular exercise in our daily lives … even if you don't have a pound to lose!

The benefits are HUGE! In addition to overall better health, you'll develop a better understanding and awareness about your body. You'll also feel energetic and less stressed while acquiring more stamina and strength.

So, have you tossed your head back, rolled your eyes and recited a "YADA … YADA … YADA" about now? I understand! I really do! But facts are facts, and you just can't ignore the fact that exercise plays a vital role in overall good health and weight loss/maintenance. However, with that said, I can't say I'm a big fan of typical regimented exercise routines developed by others. While they may work for some, over time I think the success rate of sticking to them for most is very low.

Let's be honest, if you're following a regimented exercise program you really don't like for the sole purpose of losing weight, I'll bet once you've lost weight *(if you stick with it that long)* you'll probably stop doing it altogether. Am I right?

That's why I believe each person should develop their own exercise regime with the understanding it will be something they plan to stick with long term -- for life!

After many attempts to find something I could stick with, I found going to a health club at least three times a week right after work was the only way I would exercise regularly. *Please note I underlined, "right after work". If I were to go home first, I'd never get out of the house again to get there.*

I tried working out at home in my basement. Disaster! My children were upstairs screaming for me because they needed something, or more often than not, they were fighting! Without fail, my husband was unable to find something. Someone would stop by or I'd get a phone call, etc., etc. The number of interruptions I could encounter at home were endless. But to be honest, even if there were no interruptions at all, I probably wouldn't do it regularly anyway. I know how I am! I'm just not committed enough to exercise regularly when I'm at home. I can always find an excuse not to do it. But that's me. YOU, on the other hand, may be one of those people who would rather work out at home *(or have no other choice)* and can stay committed to doing it regularly. Great! Whatever works for you is what matters!

As mentioned earlier, I make it a routine to go to the gym right after work. However, I use the word "routine" loosely as my schedule changes all the time. Sometimes I can't get there on my regular night because I have to work late or attend one of my kid's functions at school, etc., etc. The reasons vary all the time, but I expect that and understand that my schedule can and will change from day to day/week to week. I just make allowances for it. The key is to be flexible but stay on track as much as possible. If you can't work out today at your normal time, then change the time if you can. Do it earlier or later or maybe you're just not going to be able to get it in at all today. Fine, but get back on track tomorrow!

The bottom line ... you've got to MOVE to burn calories. So, find some way to exercise as often as you can and don't look for excuses not to because remember ... you're only hurting yourself!

As mentioned earlier, I believe everyone's workout routine should be a personal choice. So, suprise! I'm not going to tell you what kind of routine and/or exercises you should or shouldn't do ... that's your job! Develop your own routine. You know your schedule best and what you like *(or can at least tolerate)* and don't like by now. You also probably already know what exercises you should/should not be doing to get the results you want. But, if you're not educated in this area, then GET EDUCATED! Talk to your doctor, look on the Internet or join a health club. Take advantage of the resources around you to develop your *personalized* workout routine.

I would, however, like to offer a few suggestions. First *(and I feel this is necessary to say)*, please check with your doctor ... especially if you have not exercised at all in a long time and/or have any health issues. It's always important to get a clean bill of health first. Remember ... <u>I'm not a doctor!</u> These are just my suggestions.

Stretches—before you begin, always start with some easy, all over stretches to prepare your body for exercise.

Cardiovascular—be sure to include some type of cardiovascular exercise you're comfortable doing and will realistically do regularly. There are numerous ways to get cardio exercise, i.e., aerobics, kick boxing, speed walking, biking, jogging, swimming, stair climbing, etc. Anything like this is great! An elliptical machine *(cross between a stair climbing/cross-country skiing)* is one of my personal favorites, along with the treadmill. I especially like the elliptical because it provides a very good low impact workout *(easy on my bad knees)*, but gets my heart rate up. Start out slow *(5–10 minutes)*, and gradually work your way up to at least 30 minutes or more. *I do 40–50 minutes of cardio at each workout.*

Weights—in addition to cardio exercise, I recommend working out with weights. It can be free weights or a weight machine, whichever you prefer. Like the cardio exercise, start out slow with light weights and gradually work your way up to heavier weights. Keep in mind as you add more weight you'll build bigger muscles. So, if your goal is to just tone up, stay with the lighter weights and do more repetitions. Important, be sure you're using the weights in a slow, controlled manner. It really concerns me when I see people yanking weights up and down with no control. If you use them like this, you won't receive the full benefit of exercising with them, plus you may risk injury. Remember ... slow and controlled!

I use a variety of weight machines at the gym to work my arms and legs (averaging between 30–55 pounds, two repetitions of 15–25).

Abs—finally, incorporate some kind of "core" strengthening/abdominal exercises in your routine. These are obviously important for reducing and tightening that gut, with the added benefit of strengthening your back, if done correctly. I see many people try to do traditional crunches *(lying on their back with their hands behind their head and raising their upper body)* but they do them wrong. First of all, they don't hold their stomach in. Then they repeatedly bend their head to their chest and pull on their neck when they try to rise up, rather than slightly raising their upper body and holding it. Doing them wrong just hurts your neck and doesn't really do much for your stomach. So if you decide to do these, make sure you are doing them correctly. *Personally, I don't like the traditional crunches, so I use an abdominal machine at the gym, 50 "crunches" with 50 pounds, then 100 or more with 40 pounds, in addition to some other common abdominal exercises.*

Oh, one more thing. Please don't overdo it when you start exercising. Go slow! Use light weights! I think this is one of the biggest mistakes I see most people make when they start exercising. They exercise too much or lift weights that are too heavy right from the start and then pay the price for doing so the next 2–3 days *("no pain, no gain" theory)*. That's crazy! Overdoing it will only leave you in pain and is completely unnecessary. So, please don't do this to yourself.

Do your research. Experiment with different exercises and decide what you are comfortable doing and not doing. From there, develop your own routine. Just be sure it *challenges* you *(work up a sweat)* and includes a variety of exercises that cover all areas of your body. Keep in mind, if something is too hard initially it should become easier as you develop more strength, so stay with it and DON'T BE LAZY! By including a variety of exercises, you'll strengthen different muscle groups so you're not just working the same ones over and over again. Also, periodically change your routine to include new exercises.

I took a Pilates class once for ten weeks and really enjoyed it. Pilates is a great way to start exercising. It's low impact and helps strengthen your core in addition to a number of other benefits. For more information, do a search on the Internet for "Pilates" or call your local health club to inquire about classes.

Obviously, implementing a regular exercise routine into your life will probably require some lifestyle changes at home. So, if you have a family, I recommend having a family meeting to discuss what those changes will be. Explain how important this is to you and your health. Ask for their support. Talk about expectations and set ground rules. For instance, if they need you for something while you are in the middle of exercising, let them know what kind of response they can expect to receive. Discuss how other potential interruptions should be handled, i.e., if you receive a phone call or someone comes to the door, etc.

Thinking through these kinds of situations ahead of time and discussing how you would like them to be handled will save you and your family a lot of confusion, frustration and fighting.

Getting your family on board will not only increase your chances of success it will teach your kids *(by example)* the importance of good health.

Just remember to be realistic and flexible. Don't sabotage yourself by trying to commit to a routine that is flat out unrealistic and you know won't work long term. Our lives are hectic and schedules change quickly, so if your routine isn't somewhat flexible, over time it may become just too hard to stick with.

Thinking of joining a fitness center/gym?

Great! Do it! Don't be intimidated! When I tell people I work out at a fitness center/gym, some have commented they wouldn't feel comfortable working out at one. When I ask why, the most common response is because they think people who are members of a gym/fitness center all have perfect bodies and prance around in fashionable little workout outfits. NONSENSE! Now I can't speak for gyms in trendier parts of the country, but here in the midwest … people go to the gym to work out, not make a fashion statement!

Hopefully, I've convinced you of the importance of this commitment and you're ready to get started. But if you're still not convinced, then all I can say is, if you are not willing to make an effort to exercise regularly in some capacity, I don't believe you are truly ready and/or committed yet to do what it takes to lose weight and develop a healthy lifestyle. Forgive me for being blunt, but you may still be looking for the lazy way out and/or for someone or something else to fix your problem.

Remember: THERE IS NO MAGIC PILL!

Losing weight and successfully keeping it off requires commitment and dedication to change the *lifestyle* that got you here in the first place. This is not a temporary situation just until you lose weight. Your overall chances of losing weight and successfully keeping it off over time are severely limited if you don't include regular exercise in your life.

COME ON! Exercise doesn't have to be torture! Pick something fun, or at the very least, tolerable to get started with. Skiing, ice skating, roller skating, dancing/aerobics, etc., are all fun activities. By choosing something fun in the begining it will help get you started and getting started is half the battle anyway, right? After that, keeping your motivation will probably be your next biggest challenge. So here are a few ideas to help with that.

Keeping your motivation:

1. If you work out at home, schedule your workouts during the same time a regular favorite television show comes on. T.V. can help reduce boredom and help you create a routine. Read a favorite book while walking on the treadmill, riding a stationary bike, etc.

2. Listen to your favorite music CD or watch music videos. *(Those skinny girls and buff guys in music videos should help give you some incentive).*

3. Recruit a workout buddy. A friend can really help keep you motivated and accountable.

4. Pictures. Cut out a picture of a sexy dress, swim suit, etc., something you'd really love to see you rself wear when you reach your goal weight. Or if it applies, how about digging out an old picture of yourself when you were thin? Carry these pictures with you and refer to them when you're feeling weak and/or losing focus and need some incentive and willpower.

5. Visualization. **A great motivator!** While exercising, visualize yourself at your goal weight in different situations. Here's my favorite: Vacationing on a hot, sunny tropical beach, stretched out on a big lounge chair, wearing a sexy bikini *(one I actually look decent in)*, enjoying a tall, cold margarita as a cool gentle ocean breeze lightly passes over my hot, svelt, tanned body. Ahhhh! Get the "picture"?

    Upcoming events can also be great motivators. Visualize yourself looking fantastic at the holidays, a family wedding, class reunion or running into an ex-boyfriend/girlfriend. But remember, only positive images, nothing negative.

6. If you have kids, get them involved! Kids love to be included in things we do and it will help teach them the importance of good health. Buy an aerobic/dance DVD designed for kids. This will keep them busy while you do your exercise, or better yet, find one you can all do together.

So, what do you do when you just can't seem to get motivated to exercise on a particular day?

Oh, those lazy days! Boy, do I have my share of them! I can come up with some great excuses to justify not exercising, "I've had such a long day and I'm just too tired. I deserve a break!" or "It's my 'time of the month' and I feel too crappy to work out." While I have to fight to stay disciplined sometimes, I'm always entertained by others excuses for never exercising.

The most popular ... "I just don't have time".

Listen ... I'm a wife, mother of two teenage children, work a full-time job, have laundry, dishes, house cleaning, cooking, yard work, kids' functions to attend, etc., etc.. All the same responsibilities as a lot of people and perhaps more than some people, but I find time to fit it in somewhere. I may have to exercise less one week or maybe not at all, change my regular work out time and/or day, or just have enough time to do a quick work out, etc. But I do my best to fit it in somewhere, somehow, constantly reminding myself ... doing SOMETHING, is better than doing NOTHING at all.

It comes down to setting priorities. If you make exercise a priority, you'll generally find time to do it. I bet most of us can usually "find time" to plop down on the couch at night and watch a sporting event or favorite television show, right? Well, it's because you've made that a priority and that's okay. My point is, instead of just sitting on your butt watching it, why not walk on a treadmill or ride a stationary bike while watching it?

The truth is we all have lazy days. You'll just have to find your own way to overcome them.

I use a guilt tactic. Seriously! I know it may sound funny, but I actually do this. Deep down I know exercising is one of the best things I can do for myself *(physically and mentally)* and I know I will feel better about it once I'm there. So, this forces me to admit I'm just being lazy and I don't really have a good excuse to skip it. Other times, I'll negotiate the intensity of my workout, i.e., "I'll go, but just do cardio today". For me, half the battle is just getting there anyway. So, if I can at least get in the building, I almost always have a good full workout and leave feeling good for going. This usually works ... but not always.

If you do give in and decide not to exercise on a given day, don't beat yourself up over it. Just make a promise to get back on track tomorrow, but then DO IT! And don't allow yourself to get in the habit of doing this often.

I can assure you, if you make the effort to exercise, it won't take long to reap the rewards, both physically and mentally. Believe it or not, you may even reach the point where you will miss it when you don't work out. Really!

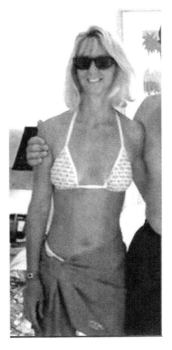

This picture was taken in Cancun. My husband and I were there celebrating our 10th wedding anniversary. I was 37 years old.

To weigh or not to weigh ... that is the question!

Deciding when you should weigh yourself and how often can differ depending on who you talk to. I believe most people would agree weighing yourself first thing in the morning is the best time. Deciding how often seems to vary. For me, it depends on whether I'm trying to lose a couple pounds or not. I always weigh myself in the morning, but if I'm trying to lose weight I may weigh myself everyday or every other day. Otherwise, it may be once a week. I suggest you weigh yourself at least every other day after implementing your new lifestyle changes as you will receive important feedback on how your body is responding to those new changes. Think of your scale as a weight loss "tool", not your enemy. Don't get frazzled if the numbers on the scale fluctuate some. Your body will need time to adjust and you can expect to see minor fluctuations in your weight from time to time anyway. So, relax!

"HEALTHY CITIZENS ARE THE GREATEST ASSET ANY COUNTRY CAN HAVE"
—*Winston Churchill*

7

Today

Well, I must admit there were times over the course of writing this when I felt like such a hypocrite and contemplated whether I should even continue. I mean … here I was preaching about eating healthy, etc., and I just crammed down several cookies and a glass of milk!

But, the more I thought about it, the more convinced I became that's exactly why I should write it … because I'm NORMAL! Yes, I give in to cravings now and then and no, I don't always eat healthy 24/7. With my lifestyle it would be unrealistic to think I could. But I was still able to lose weight and keep it off and under control all these years, even after two pregnancies and while going through menopause. So, I know you can do it too. Just stay focused and committed to your overall goal of <u>good health,</u> physically and spiritually.

So, what do I do today *(20 years later)* to maintain my weight? Well, I use the same basic principles I've always used.

I eat very lean meat, fish, and chicken prepared grilled or baked (I love grilled salmon). Fruits, vegetables, pasta and only whole grain bread *(limit or eliminate carbohydrates at dinner if trying to lose weight)*.

I limit fatty foods like butter sauces, mayonnaise, fast food, soda and junk food. I routinely avoid fried foods and rich, heavy sauces, like alfredo.

I also pay attention to balance and portion sizes.

Again, it's okay to have that cookie or ice cream cone once in a while as long as you eat the good stuff most of the time. Equally important is paying attention to portion sizes. Don't pile your plate up with loads of food, even if they are healthy. Learn to eat less. I like to follow the principle, eat light, but often. I believe eating small amounts throughout the day is a good way to keep your metabolism in good working order and energy levels up, plus it helps keep your appetite under control. But again … as long as you choose the right foods!

Choosing the right foods will be a lot easier if you're prepared. Don't put yourself in a situation where you're "forced" to resort to that donut or bag of microwave popcorn and soda to satisfy your hunger. Pack your lunches and snacks for the day so you have healthy food readily available to reduce/eliminate temptation to grab something unhealthy.

Below is an example of what I would typically eat in a day during the week.

Morning: A cup or two of coffee *(No, it's not decaffeinated either, I need caffeine!)* Most often, oatmeal or dry cereal around 10:00/10:30 a.m., if I'm hungry.

Afternoon: I almost always bring my lunch to work. Frozen lunches: Lean Cuisine/Kashi meals or I may have a salad with turkey, grilled chicken, or salmon, and lots of veggies. Sometimes it may be a Subway sandwich *(turkey or chicken breast on honey oat bread, no cheese, all veggies, and brown mustard)* and I almost always have water to drink.

Mid/late afternoon: Occasionally, an orange, banana or other fruit, a couple pretzels. Sometimes, it may a piece of chocolate, but a piece or two … not a box or a whole candy bar.

Dinner: Most often it's a serving of lean meat, *(pork, chicken, fish, 95% fat-free free hamburger, beef, etc.)* and a small portion of carbohydrates *(potatoes, noodles, etc., unless pasta happens to be the main course).* However, as I mentioned before, if I'm trying to lose a couple pounds, I may eliminate the carbohydrate items altogether at dinner and just stick to meat and vegetables. I always have at least one veggie, but sometimes two or more, water to drink or maybe a glass of wine, if we are having steak or pasta.

Evening snack: I usually don't snack in the evening, but every now and then I may have a frozen sugar-free fruit bar, or something along that line. *I try not to eat anything after 7:30/8:00 p.m.*

Exercise, of course, still plays an important role in my life. I try to work out 2–3 days a week.

Mentally/spiritually, I do what I can to maintain a positive attitude and a grateful state of mind. I take time every day to recognize and appreciate the wonderful "gifts" in my life, the ability to SEE a beautiful sunrise/sunset, to HEAR birds sing, to FEEL the warmth of the sun on a summer day, to be blessed with a loving and supportive family, awesome friends and good health. It may sound corny but it's important to me to feel good … happy! So, I plan outings/events often and spend time with family/friends doing the things I enjoy.

I am grateful not only for the things I have in my life today, but for the things yet to come. I truly do feel blessed!!

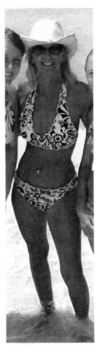

This picture was taken on the beach in Panama City Beach, Florida, June 2007. I'm two months away from my 47th birthday and weighed 116 pounds.

8

Tips/Tricks

As promised, here are some tips/tricks I used and still use today to help me lose/maintain my weight. Some will be a recap of things already mentioned in earlier chapters, but others will be new. Hopefully, you will find them as helpful as I have. Maybe they will even inspire you to come up with a few of your own.

Tips

1. ***First and foremost, make a verbal commitment "out loud" that you will start taking steps to improve your overall health (mind, body and soul).*** Unless you have some physical or mental condition beyond your control, there is no reason why you shouldn't. Write this commitment down and recite it daily.

2. ***Take a daily multi-vitamin.***

3. ***One day at a time.*** Don't focus on the "mountain" *(total amount of weight you want to lose)*, set small, even daily goals to achieve. For example, in addition to my regular workout today, I'm going to take a walk and ensure I don't eat anything after 7:00/7:30 p.m. Concentrate on getting through one day at a time. You didn't gain the weight overnight so understand you are not realistically going to lose it overnight either. Practice patience!

4. ***It doesn't have to be all or nothing.*** Just because you "lost it" and wolfed down a half of a box of cookies is no reason to give in to a total binge or give up all together. STOP NOW! Forgive yourself for having a weak moment and get back on track.

5. ***Concentrate on what you CAN eat instead of what you can't.*** If you focus on the foods you can't eat, you'll probably feel deprived and depressed. Instead, focus on all the good, healthy food choices you do have. Remember:

you can eat anything you want ... but you're *choosing* to eat the good stuff.

6. ***Stay on track!*** Don't allow yourself to be seduced/side-tracked by weight loss advertisements. Remember, there is no magic pill or diet plan. Stop looking for one! Stay committed to your plan! If tempted to eat something you know you shouldn't, ask yourself if it's really worth it and refer to those pictures you cut out for strength.

7. ***Keep busy!*** Keeping busy will help keep your mind off food.

8. ***Get plenty of rest.*** It's important to get a good night's sleep regularly as it will help keep you physically and mentally strong to stay on track. I know when I am tired I'm more likely to eat things I wouldn't normally eat and less likely to exercise.

9. ***Motivation.*** Earlier we discussed some ways to help keep your motivation *(refer to Chapter 6).* I like planning gatherings and/or small trips regularly so I have something to look forward to.

10. ***Learn to listen to your body.*** Take time to learn about your body, paying special attention to the cycles it goes through, e.g., it can be very common for women to gain up to five pounds or so around that time of the month. Your appetite may also increase. So, don't expect to lose weight during this time or be upset because you've gained a little. This is normal for a lot of women. If you stay on track, it's most likely water weight anyway and will disappear in a couple days.

11. ***Take lessons from thin people.*** Instead of making excuses for people who are thin, why not watch, ask questions and learn from them? If you decided to play a musical instrument, speak a foreign language, or participate in a new sport, you'd probably take lessons and/or learn from others with experience, right? Well, why not use the same approach when learning how to be thin? Watch what thin people eat, how much, how often and how active they are. While there will always be exceptions, most often you'll see very distinct differences between how a thin person lives their life versus an overweight person. It just makes sense, right? So, watch, listen, ask questions, and finally take action to incorporate some of those same habits.

12. ***Visualization.*** Again this is HUGE! If you were thin in the past, post those thin pictures of yourself somewhere you can see them each day. Cut out a picture of an outfit, bathing suit, dress, etc., you'd like to wear when you've reached your goal weight and hang it somewhere you can see it regularly. Make it a daily practice to sit back, close your eyes and visualize yourself at your goal weight. Recognize how you feel during this time.

13. ***Don't purchase larger clothes to compensate for weight gained.*** If you've gained weight, <u>NEVER</u> go out and buy larger size clothes. In my opinion, you're giving yourself permission to keep the weight on and ... room to grow! Instead, take steps immediately to lose the extra weight.

14. ***Buy a cookbook on healthy, low-fat cooking and commit to try at least one new recipe each week.*** This will help prevent boredom as well as possibly introduce you to new types of food and/or cooking techniques.

15. ***Plant a garden and/or grow fresh herbs.*** Growing your own fruits, vegetables and herbs can be fun and will encourage you and your family to eat them as well as give you an opportunity to experiment cooking with a different spices. Eating items picked from your own garden is a wonderful way to appreciate their freshness and flavor. *But be warned, once you've had them this fresh it's hard to settle for anything less.*

16. ***Always look for opportunities to exercise.*** Don't just rely on your regular scheduled time to exercise. Look for other opportunities throughout the day to get exercise, e.g., take the stairs when possible, park farther out in the parking lots, walk or ride a bike to work, go for a walk on your lunch hour, etc.

17. ***Eat light, but more often.*** Eat smaller meals or snacks throughout the day instead of three large meals. But, it must be the good stuff ... no junk!

18. ***Balance and portion control.*** Reducing portion sizes in the beginning was tough for me since I was used to eating more. So, to help curb my ravenous appetite, I occasionally took half of a diet pill (or half a dose) to help me stay in control. Occasionally I would also take them for a day or two around that "time of the month" to help curb my ravenous appetite. But, please understand I didn't make a habit of this and by no means am I suggesting you take these. I'm just explaining what I did. I highly recommend you check with your doctor first if you decide to take these, especially if you have any health

conditions and/or taking other medications, etc. Remember, I'm not a doctor!

19. ***Eat the majority of carbohydrate foods during the day, limit or eliminate them at dinner time.*** Try to eat the majority of any carbohydrates during the day when you are more active. Eat small portions, or eliminate them all together at dinner time. Replace potatoes, noodles, rice, etc., with more vegetables.

20. ***Dealing with mid-afternoon cravings.*** Sometime around 3:00 p.m., I get hit with a mid-afternoon craving *(or boredom, I'm not always sure which one it really is)*. To satisfy my craving and avoid grabbing quick fix junk food, I bring an apple, banana, or dried fruit, *(something healthy)* to eat. This helps take the late afternoon edge off without resorting to junk food, and helps prevent snacking before dinner.

Tricks

Satisfying a sweet tooth

By now you may have read or heard the best way to deal with a craving for sweets is to "wait it out", until the craving passes. While I do believe this is true, if you can do it, great! But this usually doesn't work for me. I generally crave something sweet right after a meal and waiting for the craving to pass can sometimes be torture. So, rather than fighting the craving, I looked for a way to satisfy it without totally sabotaging myself. Below are a few things I may eat or drink to help take take the edge off:

- Very small glass of diet pop/root beer or sugar-free lemonade
- A few sugar free mints
- Piece of sugar-free hard candy or gum
- Serving of dried fruit
- Small serving of sugar-free Jello with a little non-fat whipped cream
- A frozen sugar-free fruit bar
- A glass of low-fat chocolate soy milk
- Sometimes, I just give in and eat a piece of chocolate!

Late night snacking

Obviously, we all know we should avoid doing this at all cost. Realistically, however, there are those times when you just feel you have to have something. So, try one of these:

- Hot beverages can help make you feel full and possibly curb a craving. Try diet hot chocolate or decaffeinated flavored tea.

- Plain popcorn or frozen sugar-free fruit bar.

- *BEST:* Brush your teeth! Yes, this can work. You'll be less likely to eat something if you know you'll have to brush your teeth again before bed.

Prevent over-eating when you arrive home

On your way home after a long day, many of us may arrive still stressed from the day and HUNGRY. To satisfy our hunger *(or reaction to stress)* we tend to grab anything quick and easy to stuff in our mouths. As discussed earlier, you can avoid this by being prepared with healthy, easy-to-grab snacks readily available. Here are a couple other things you can also try to help control this before you get home:

- Drink a bottle of water (preferably) or a can of diet pop on your way home. This will help fill you up enough so you'll feel in control when you arrive.

- Visualization. Close your eyes and visualize exactly what you're going to do when you walk through that door. What healthy snack will you grab or what will you do to keep yourself busy until dinner? By taking time to visually plan ahead, you'll feel more in control when you arrive and you'll make better choices.

Eating out in Restaurants

Try to pick restaurants that offer a variety of food as well as preparation methods. Avoid items that are breaded or fried, always stick with foods that are baked, steamed, grilled or broiled.

- Ask to have all sauces/dressings served on the side, e.g., salad dressings. Instead of pouring the dressing all over your salad, gently dip every other bite into it, tapping off excess. Work to reach the point where you're eating more salad without dressing than with dressing. I eat less than a quarter of the dressing served this way.

- Order extra vegetables in place of mashed potatoes, rice, pasta, etc. If you do have a baked potato, order it without the butter and sour cream. If you just can't eat it plain, try putting vegetables on top of it, or order some fat free ranch dressing or low fat sour cream and dip every other bite in it, the same way you would your salad.

Parties

If there is a table full of appetizers, it's okay to have a few, but …

- Choose the ones that are good for you, i.e. veggies (avoid dips), fruit, pretzels or a few whole grain crackers, etc.

- Don't stand and/or socialize next to the snack table. Move as far away from it as possible. You'll be less likely to eat as much if you have to make a conscious effort to walk over to it to get food each time.

- Socialize—it will help keep your mind off food.

- Limit alcohol consumption—it will also help prevent the urge to stop at your favorite fast food restaurant late at night when you're driving home.

Well, I guess that about wraps it up! I suppose I should apologize if you were hoping to read about some new "miracle" method for losing weight. But, as you've read, the methods I use and advocate are basically simple …

"Create an environment and lifestyle that promotes and encourages a healthy <u>mind</u>, <u>body</u> and <u>spirit</u> and you will succeed at anything, including losing weight and keeping it off."

I sincerely hope you've found this information beneficial. I recommend reading this guide again and refer to it often to help maintain your focus.

I wish you much success in achieving your goal of a happy, healthy new lifestyle and remember …

"WHATEVER THE MIND OF MAN CAN CONCEIVE AND BELIEVE, IT CAN ACHIEVE!"

YOU CAN DO THIS!

www.IFinallyUnderstand.com

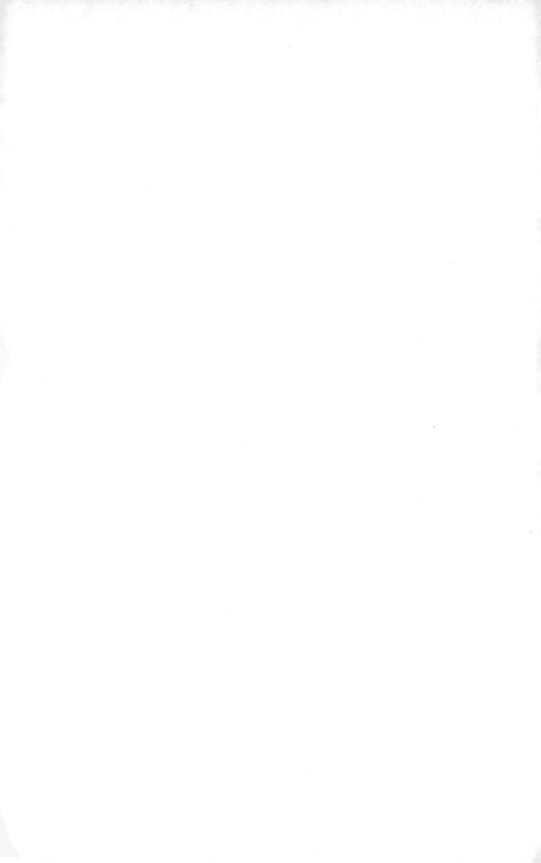

LaVergne, TN USA
01 June 2010
184559LV00004BA/46/P